HEATHER DOLSON

A Path to Wholeness

Journal Prompts and Affirmations for Coping with Pregnancy Loss

First published by Heather on Health 2022

Copyright © 2022 by Heather Dolson

All rights reserved. No part of this publication may be reproduced, stored or transmitted in any form or by any means, electronic, mechanical, photocopying, recording, scanning, or otherwise without written permission from the publisher. It is illegal to copy this book, post it to a website, or distribute it by any other means without permission.

Heather Dolson asserts the moral right to be identified as the author of this work.

Heather Dolson has no responsibility for the persistence or accuracy of URLs for external or third-party Internet Websites referred to in this publication and does not guarantee that any content on such Websites is, or will remain, accurate or appropriate.

Designations used by companies to distinguish their products are often claimed as trademarks. All brand names and product names used in this book and on its cover are trade names, service marks, trademarks and registered trademarks of their respective owners. The publishers and the book are not associated with any product or vendor mentioned in this book. None of the companies referenced within the book have endorsed the book.

First edition

This book was professionally typeset on Reedsy. Find out more at reedsy.com

*This is dedicated to my mom,
the first woman who shared her stories of pregnancy loss with me.*

Contents

1	Introduction	1
2	Acknowledge the Loss	9
3	Making Space for Grief	13
4	Loving Support	17
5	Navigating Relationships	21
6	Wholesome Body	26
7	Mental Health Care	30
8	Releasing Shame and Guilt	35
9	Moving Forward	39
10	Conclusion	43
11	Resources	46

1

Introduction

To begin I want to say I am so sorry for your loss. I can only imagine the pain you are feeling right now.

While we all have different stories and paths in life, as human beings the pain of loss, grief, sadness, and anger are universal emotions that we can all relate to, no matter the situation or circumstance.

My professional background is one of a nurse and coach. In my 14-year nursing career, I have experienced so much death and dying as the natural process of life. I have been able to support families and loved ones of dying patients and help people die with dignity, love, and support. It has been a privilege.

I am passionate about reducing stigma around taboo subjects such as mental health. Mental health was my first love and niche in my nursing career and one I hold very close to my heart and in my continued coaching work.

My own personal journey led me to yoga and meditation nearly 20 years ago. I have experienced the profound effects of this practice in my life and how it has anchored me in difficult times. My background in yoga and meditation has influenced these pages and the soul work that I'm inviting you to do now.

With your pregnancy loss, you may have had an early miscarriage, a late miscarriage, medical termination, or maybe you saw your baby born but he or she never had their chance to take their first breath of life.

My heart aches for you.

I have 2 babies and I remember my pregnancies with both of them like it was yesterday. I remember the fear of losing them. I remember being scared if I didn't feel kicks. I remember the profound overwhelm with the first heartbeat. I know that you attach and become a mother at the moment of conception and you would do anything to love and protect your baby from that moment forward.

At the moment of conception, your hearts connected, your souls aligned, your energies intertwined. Your baby's soul chose you as its mother to carry it for however long you did.

As a coach, spiritual mentor, and personal development enthusiast, I created this guide to support you lovingly and deeply through this difficult journey to wholeness.

I know it is hard to believe right now, but you can feel whole again.

I know you may feel empty right now.

I know you can feel happiness again.

INTRODUCTION

I know you can feel joy.

You deserve to be in all of your wholeness, and have all the love, joy and happiness that is your birthright.

In this book I have included practical tools such as journal prompts and affirmations so that you can empower yourself and tap into your own unique healing and wisdom.

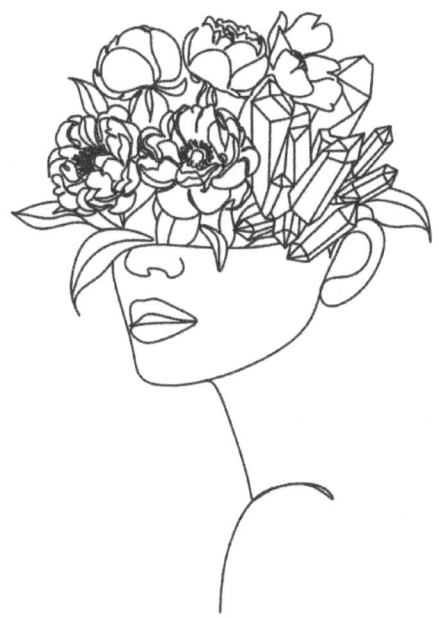

JOURNALING PRACTICE

Along my journey of personal growth and spiritual evolution, if there is one thing I have struggled with it has been consistency with journaling or just sitting down and doing it! That is like so many habits in life that take time to develop and become a part of you.

Half of the battle is carving out the time to show up and sit down and do it. This is true for most habits that are healthy and whole, whether it's exercise, healthy eating, meditation, creative outlets.

Self-discipline is the deepest form of self-love. Self discipline is not a negative thing. It's not authoritarian. Self discipline is realizing your value so greatly that you prioritize focused time and loving actions for yourself.

Journaling and free flow writing without judgment and self-editing is one of the best ways to gain emotional awareness and grow personally. The truth is you are your own best teacher and healer, and guided journaling can be a transformative process.

Research has shown that writing about your personal feelings can decrease anxiety and your perception of stress in tough times. Journaling has been shown to increase personal resilience and social integration (Smyth et al., 2018). Social isolation is widely discussed as a struggle for so many women and partners who suffer pregnancy loss.

When a person journals even twice a week, it can reduce anxiety and depression significantly (Smyth et al., 2018).

The other benefits of journaling are that you don't have to see anybody to do it and can practice this in the comfort of your own home. Psychological support from a professional is strongly recommended

INTRODUCTION

in this time of loss and grief. However, professional support is not always feasible or accessible to many women or their partners. There are so many barriers to this care such as cost, lack of insurance, and the attached stigma (Smyth et al., 2018).

Journaling is cost-efficient and a pen and paper is easily accessible to almost anyone.

So if it's so easily accessible, why is it so hard to stick with something like journaling?

Journaling may not always be comfortable emotionally because it involves sitting down and tuning in to your feelings, which can be a scary place to go sometimes. There is that saying though, if you don't feel it, you don't heal it.

Repressing emotions will cause them to be stored in our bodies, creating pain, tension, and stored trauma. They have to go somewhere! They get bottled up and the pressure increases. It can lead to depression and other mental health struggles. These repressed emotions can explode out at inopportune times with loved ones or in other situations where it's not the appropriate time or place for that expression. Journaling provides a healthy outlet and a black and white method to get all of the emotions and thoughts out of you and express it in a tangible way.

On another level, journaling can create some detachment. With time you can see patterns, repetitive thoughts, and very much like an objective observer, you can create some space from it and gain more self awareness.

Here are a few tips for developing a journal practice:

1. Try to journal every day, even if it's for 5 minutes. If words are not coming to you, then draw or doodle. Make it a practice and commitment to yourself to create this time and space just for you. Set a timer and then stop looking at the clock.
2. Start the practice by tuning in to yourself. Take 3 deep breaths. Put your hand on your heart and set an intention to allow yourself to express freely without judgment.
3. Use an old fashioned pen and paper as there is something very powerful about this act of physically writing. It's not wrong to type it on your computer notes, but play around with this and see how each method feels.
4. Just let the words flow. Don't think about grammar or how it sounds. Don't be rigid about it. Use your journal time when it works for you. If you do start judging yourself, let it go and return to writing. This is a mindfulness practice in itself.
5. Finally, use the journal prompts in this book to help guide your practice. Don't feel like you have to use all of them. Pick the ones that resonate or stick out to you. Trust your internal guidance system. You are your best healer.

Affirmations

Affirmations are words that are uplifting and positive. When they are repeated they can help in re-programming our minds from the usual default negative thought patterns and habitual programming that is our conditioning from childhood and previous generations.

The repetition of affirmations is a way to redirect your mind to a new thought; one that is more uplifting and empowering.

INTRODUCTION

Affirmations are similar to *mantras*. As a yogi, I love the use of mantra or yoga sounds. For the purpose of this book, the focus will be on written word affirmations.

Repeating affirmations can be an interesting practice. You may not resonate with the words right away. You may say it and not believe it. You may say it and it brings up feelings of denial, anger, disbelief, discomfort, anxiety. That's okay.

I encourage you to pick an affirmation in this book - one or two, and there are several to choose from. Find ways to make it more familiar. Again, be flexible and flow. You can change your affirmations and let your intuition guide you.

The important thing for integration is to find creative ways to make it a part of your daily life.

Write the affirmations on your mirror. Schedule reminders in your phone. Put it on your screensaver. Say it out loud. Keep it close to you at the beginning, written on a note in your pocket. Say it while looking at yourself in the mirror. Write them down in your journal and let it flow there.

- How does it feel in your body when you say the affirmation?
- Where do you feel it in your body?
- Do you feel any resistance to the words? Where do you feel this?
- What is the root of this resistance?
- What is the conflicting thought or belief to the affirmation?
- Can you remember an experience that may have led you to believe the opposite of the affirmation?

I strongly recommend taking ideas from this book to shape your own unique affirmation in words that resonate with you. This is even more powerful!

The power of *mantras* or elevating words of affirmations is the ability to cut off a negative thought or you can think of it as pruning the vine in gardening. When you realize you are circling around in a negative and toxic cycle, just stop, don't judge yourself, prune the vine, and repeat your affirmation. The more you do this, the more you create new patterns of thinking. This is active meditation!

See if you can take it a step further and get into the emotion and feeling associated with the affirmation. Use your imagination for this. Visualize a scene or conversation to evoke this emotion. Really allow yourself and your body and your mind to get into the imagination and energy of the feeling and say the words of affirmation.

Notice how you feel when you cultivate the emotional energy with the words.

There is no right or wrong way to do this, only a willingness and an open heart.

Without further ado, I bring you to the first part of the book and an important first step...acknowledging the loss.

2

Acknowledge the Loss

Pregnancy loss is so difficult, devastating, and isolating. You may have loving support in your life. You may not have a lot of support, which emphasizes that feeling of loneliness. Many people just may not know what to say to comfort you. Every situation is different.

People struggle with grief and there is added stigma attached to pregnancy loss. For example, you likely see or hear an outpouring of condolences when someone's father dies.

Generally words of comfort and condolences are not shared and expressed as openly with pregnancy loss as it may not be perceived as a "socially acceptable" death, for lack of a better term. This is for a variety of reasons.

Grief is so complex and experienced individually.

With early miscarriage, maybe you hadn't told anyone for fear of the risk of losing the baby. This is an old tradition - not to tell anyone before 16 weeks of pregnancy. This further perpetuates the feelings of isolation and stigma of loss. So you may be suffering the loss in silence.

That may not have been the case and you told as many people as you could about your pregnancy because you were so excited or far along in your pregnancy.

Your baby might have been past 20 weeks when you lost him or her or still born. In all cases of pregnancy loss, some people may acknowledge the loss with love and support while others say hurtful words, which were well meaning, and some may not say anything at all.

Some things you hear that are not helpful are:

Everything happens for a reason.

It was for the best.

Nature takes care of things.

You can always have another one.

Wait until you're married.

I want you to know it is a *real* loss at whatever stage you lost your baby. You are allowed to feel everything you feel. You alone can acknowledge the loss as this is the most important place the acknowledgment comes from on your journey.

Use the following journal prompts to explore your inner world and emotions as you grieve. Remember you are brave and you are strong. I believe you can get through this.

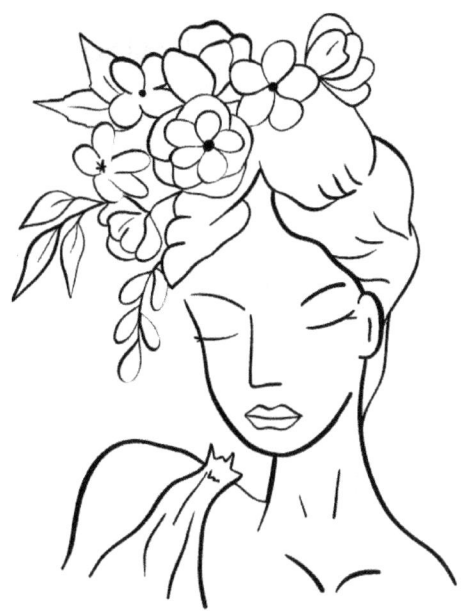

Journal Prompts

When I lost my baby it felt like this…

When I lost my baby this is what was going through my head…

Today, I'm having a hard time with…

When I'm sad, I feel it in my body like this…

I feel angry about…

Here are 3 ways I can be compassionate with myself today...

If I was an outsider responding to myself and the loss I just experienced, this is what I would do or say to comfort myself...

If I could have said goodbye to my baby, this is what I would have said...

Write about 1 difficult thing in your life that you accept? How did you get to that point of acceptance?

Affirmations

In my sadness, I still love and accept myself.

It is safe to be me.

It is safe to feel all the feelings flowing through me.

Losing my baby was a real loss and no one else needs to understand it completely.

It's okay to mourn, but I will not lose myself.

It's okay to be angry at losing my baby.

It's okay to be angry with God.

I allow myself to be present and feel fully.

It's okay to feel relief.

3

Making Space for Grief

Grief is like the ocean, it comes in waves ebbing and flowing. Sometimes the water is calm, and sometimes it is overwhelming. All we can do is learn to swim.
~ Vicki Harrison

Grief is a complex emotion - it's vast and undefined, ever changing, and comes in waves. Each person experiences grief uniquely and there really is no right or wrong way. Give yourself the time and space to grieve. Take time away from work. Carve out physical and energetic space alone to allow the space and time for all the feelings to flow through you. If you have a partner, maybe this is something you can do together as well.

Loss is part of the human experience - one we all will go through.

Pregnancy loss can fall under *disenfranchised grief*.

What does this mean?

This is when your support system or community does not acknowledge your loss as legitimate. This can be the case with other situations like job loss, a move, losing a pet. A person may have significant grief with these situations, but external sources basically view the grief as socially unacceptable (*What Is Disenfranchised Grief?*, 2022).

This can make your grief experience incredibly challenging.

Anytime you hear yourself saying "I shouldn't feel this way" come to this book and use the tools in this book.

Grief is a process and multi-dimensional. Elizabeth Kübler Ross is well known for her work with death and grief and her book *Death and Dying* (*EKR Foundation, 2020*). She explored 5 stages of grief in her work:

1. Denial
2. Anger
3. Bargaining
4. Depression
5. Acceptance

These stages do not happen in a particular, linear order. You can go back and forth between these common stages of grief and there is no timeline.

You may withdraw, you may want support. You may process your loss entirely differently. These 5 stages of grief are simply a guide. You can keep them in mind as you approach the following journal prompts to support your grieving process.

Journal Prompts

Where do I feel grief in my body? Where does my grief stay?

Today, I miss…

A feeling I've felt a lot lately is…

If I could tell my baby something, this would be it…

I can honor my baby by doing these 3 things…

When do I feel the most sadness? What does sadness feel like for me?

Write a letter to your baby.

Write a letter to yourself.

Write a letter to anyone else. (You don't have to send it).

Affirmations

I allow all the feelings to flow through me today.

It's okay to take time and space to grieve.

I'm moving through grief today and onto other emotions.

I am strong and can embrace my grief.

Recovery takes time and I heal at my own pace.

Each day I can choose to release some sadness and grief.

Tears are a natural release of anger and sadness.

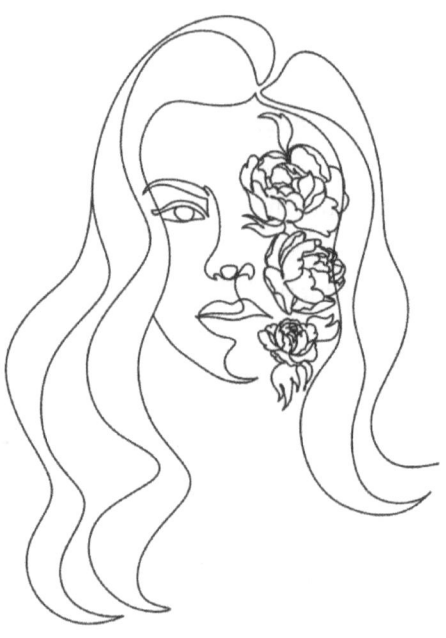

4

Loving Support

You are surrounded by love and support from the Universe, God, Spirit, Source, Mother Earth. You can call it whatever you like. Maybe you don't have those beliefs and that is okay. I have a feeling if you have discovered this book and it's already in your hands…you have some kind of belief in Higher Power outside or within yourself.

You can be a pillar of support for yourself in this time because you are supported by these invisible forces if you realize it and open your heart to it.

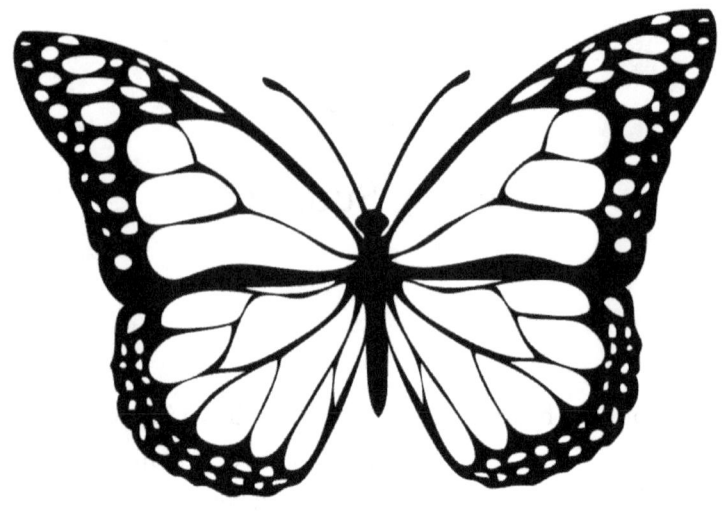

No matter what your situation or circumstance, single or attached, supportive family or friends or lack thereof - you never have to be alone in it all. In practical terms, you may need to seek out a counselor, therapist, medical professional, or grief coach. It's okay to ask for help and loving support. As a single mom, I know that asking for help can be a block sometimes. Some of us feel we have to be strong and persevere and do it all on our own; that it's weak to ask for help.

It takes courage and strength to ask for help.

If you have barriers to seeking external help, journaling is accessible to you right now. You rely on yourself. You make the space and time available. All you need to do is sit and write.

Journal Prompts

Does it feel uncomfortable asking for help? Where do you feel it in your body?

I need more of...

I need less of...

I am willing to let go of...

I am willing to release...

What is one thing you could try to make easier on yourself today...

How are you supported right now?

List 3 sources of support right now, seen or unseen.

Is there anyone else I know going through this right now? How can we support each other?

Affirmations

I choose love.

I deserve to be supported and I am open to receiving that support.

I am surrounded by love and support.

I am not alone.

I live in the present to heal my past.

I'm surrounded by support, seen and unseen.

The universe supports and guides me. (Feel free to replace the Universe with God, Angels, Spirit, Divine Power, Source).

5

Navigating Relationships

Pregnancy loss can strain close relationships or it can bring you closer together. This applies to relationships with partners, spouses, family, friends.

Grief is an individual journey and people process it differently. This is what can make it difficult to relate to the ones closest; for example, if your partner just doesn't seem to understand the loss or seems ambivalent. Whether you have a spouse or you are single, I hope you have someone in your life you can confide in.

As a single mom, I especially hope this book is inclusive for all women, single or attached.

These relationship conflicts can arise in different ways with your parent, sibling, or friend. There may be conflict because these people don't seem supportive or understand your grief.

For the purpose of this section, the term "support person" will cover all personal relationships such as spouse, partner, parent, sibling, friend, co-worker and to provide all-inclusive language.

Journal Prompts

Write down a list of people you can turn to for support, either in person or virtually.

I feel most connected to my support person when…

If you could tell your support person about your day, what would you tell them?

How did your support person make you feel today?

What is something you wish your support person would understand?

What is something you wish your support person could help you with.

When I feel upset, I can call…

If I could tell my support person the truth, this would be it…

Is there anyone you would like to spend less time with?

If someone says something hurtful, this is how I can respond…

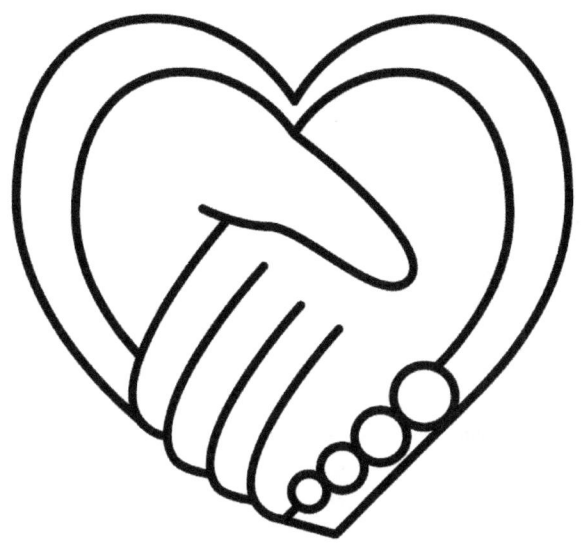

Affirmations

I give and receive love today.

I turn to love instead of loss.

I can accept help when it's offered.

I am grateful for the love and support in my life.

Love is everywhere.

I open my heart to the love around me.

I see you.

I see myself with unconditional love.

I honor you as I honor myself.

Single

Even on my own, I am already whole.

I am enough just as I am.

I got this!

I am strong and capable and I will get through this.

We all fall down in life. I stumble and get back up every time.

I will carry on.

I am doing the best with what I know right now.

I am a person who deserves to be loved.

I love and accept myself right now.

Attached

NAVIGATING RELATIONSHIPS

I look for ways to laugh with my partner.

I listen to my partner before responding in anger.

I understand that getting through the hard times will be worth it.

I decide to love my spouse each day.

I give my partner space to be an individual. We can be different and grow together.

I forgive my spouse.

I support my spouse.

I am grateful for my spouse.

6

Wholesome Body

The truth is your body is amazing. You may not feel like it right now. Your body has just gone through a birthing process at whatever stage you lost your baby. You're left with the discomfort, heavy bleeding, cramping, and no baby.

Your body hasn't failed. There is nothing wrong with you. Now more than ever, give your body the love, kindness, and compassion it craves. Know and trust that your womb is filled with wisdom. Nurture and give your body loving care as you heal.

Take time to rest and move your body mindfully. Take walks in nature. Feel your breath move in your chest. All of these practices can help bring you to the present moment.

WHOLESOME BODY

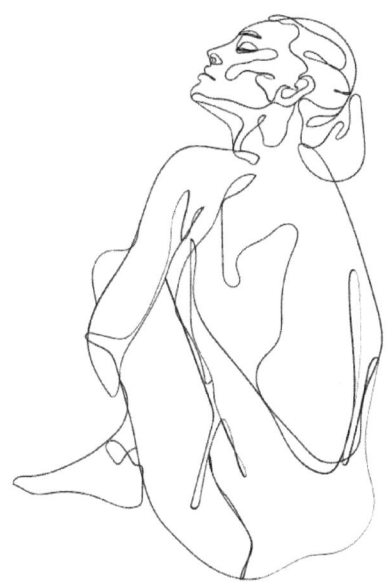

Journal Prompts

How does my body feel today?

My body does this for me…

3 loving things I can do for my body today are…

I nurture my body by doing…

What parts of my body do I find difficult to accept?

Create a nightly routine that could improve your sleep.

Can you remember a time that a negative comment was made about your body? What was it? Who said it? How did it make you feel? Do you think it sticks with you today?

List 10 things you appreciate about your body.

How do you like to move your body?

Write about a time your body protected you.

What judgments do you place on your body?

What is your current relationship with exercise?

My body changed in this way…

I want to feel like this in my body…

Affirmations

I rest when I need to.

My body is amazing.

My body deserves love and respect.

I love my body exactly as it is right now.

I am beautiful.

WHOLESOME BODY

My body is perfect exactly as it is and I honor it.

I love and trust my body.

My womb is the perfect vessel for life.

I am aware of the creative power of my womb.

I nourish my body with clean, whole foods.

My womb functions perfectly and knows exactly what it's doing.

I allow myself plenty of sleep.

My body cleanses itself as my womb cycles.

7

Mental Health Care

Pregnancy loss is devastating and impacts emotional and mental health and well-being. Sadness can lead to depression. You may have no motivation to get up, no appetite, insomnia, general apathy, decreased concentration or focus.

You may have fear about the future if you can conceive again, fear of losing the baby again if you do, fear of having to go through this indescribable pain. This anxiety could ripple out into your everyday life. You may have a racing mind that just doesn't seem to still, emotional overwhelm, irritability, anger.

Some women suffer from post traumatic stress disorder for months or years after pregnancy loss. Always know you can seek professional help from a doctor, psychotherapist, or counselor to help navigate and provide an open channel for expression and communication.

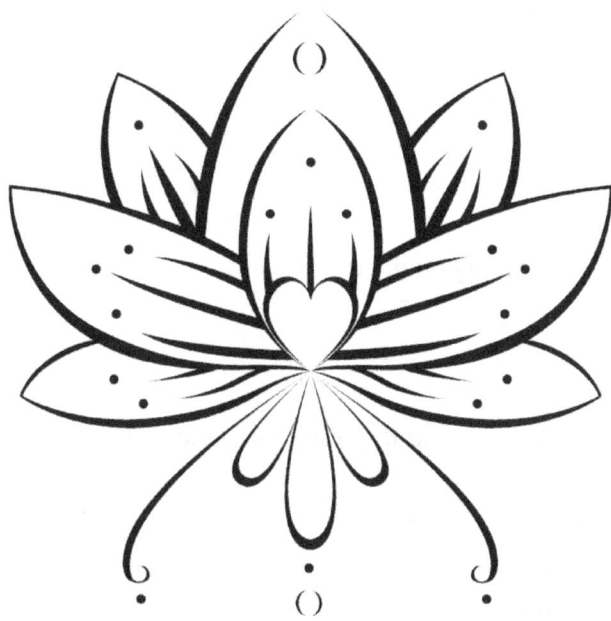

These journal prompts are intended to help you gain awareness. They are not intended to replace professional advice or support.

Journal Prompts

Where does your mind go when you let it wander?

When I'm anxious, this is how I feel it in my body...

Write a list of activities that you can engage in to make yourself feel better?

What creative ways do I use to express my feelings? If I can't think of any, what are some I can try?

I love my mind because…

What do I like about myself?

This has been weighing on my mind lately…

I fear this the most because…

What would happen if your depression went away?

Depression looks like this for me…

Depression feels like this in my body…

Affirmations

I am willing to release any negative fearful ideas from my mind, body, and life.

Wholeness is possible for me.

My diagnosis will not define my life.

I can always balance a negative thought with a positive one.

I love myself for who I am.

MENTAL HEALTH CARE

I am worthy of love, joy, and happiness.

It is safe to be me.

I have always been enough and will always be enough.

My mental health challenges do not define me.

It is possible to improve my mental health.

I am more than my trauma.

My trauma does not define me.

My feelings are valid.

I see the situation resolving for the greater good of all involved.

I am safe.

I choose to love and accept myself even though I have anxiety.

I am more than my anxious thoughts. Anxiety does not define me.

Right now I take a deep breath and I am peaceful.

There are people out there who understand what I am going through.

I am strong enough to get through this crisis.

This crisis will pass and I will be okay.

This crisis is testing me, but I am strong enough.

8

Releasing Shame and Guilt

Pregnancy is a social and developmental milestone. When women experience pregnancy loss, shame and guilt are common accompanying feelings. Women may feel that there is something wrong with them or something wrong with their bodies. They may go over and over in their head about what they could have done to prevent the loss or what they may have done that caused it. The fact is pregnancy loss happens in 1 out of 4 women. That's strikingly common. This is not meant to minimize your loss by any means, rather to give you reassurance. This is not your fault.

You are amazing. Your body is amazing. Your womb is amazing. You can let go of any shame or doubt you carry. It's simply not true.

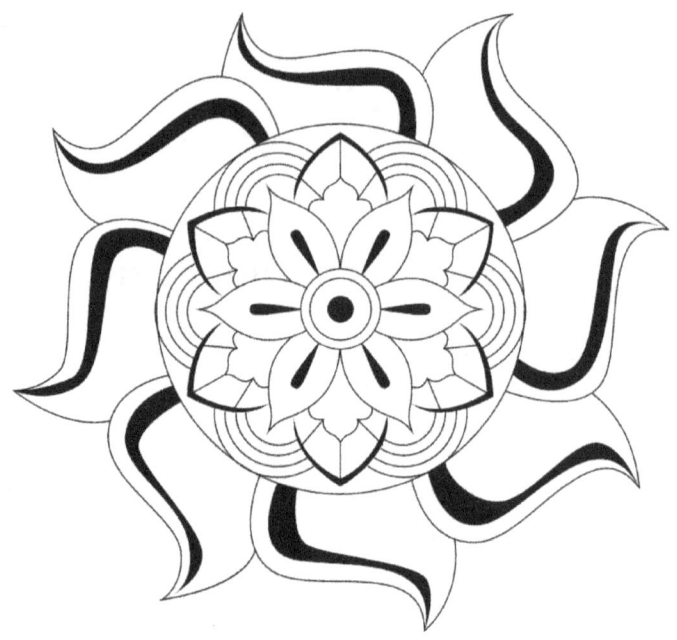

Journal Prompts

If I could forgive myself for one thing it would be…

These are things that trigger me…

How do you feel about yourself today?

Write down 3 things you have accomplished this week (even if they seem small, i.e. making the bed)…

Write a letter about what you're feeling guilty about. (You don't send it to anyone).

When was the last time you felt happy?

What last triggered feelings of shame?

What do you do when you feel shame?

Where does your guilt come from - you? Does it come from another person, a circumstance or experience?

Where do you feel shame or guilt in your body?

Who would you be if you had no shame or guilt?

Affirmations

I forgive myself.

I'm sorry. Please forgive me. Thank you. I love you.

It is safe for me to feel joy.

I release all blame and allow forgiveness to show me the way.

I release the past and it is safe for me to move forward.

I am capable of moving past this guilt.

I gently release the grip of anger from my body.

I accept that I was always doing the best I could with what I knew at the time.

A PATH TO WHOLENESS

I have the courage to become whole again.

I choose to love all of myself.

I am capable of feeling peace with the past.

When I forgive myself, I can forgive others.

I release the stories that keep me small.

9

Moving Forward

The last section was about releasing shame and guilt because this is a significant part that can hold you back from moving on.

When you are grieving, you can start to identify with these strong emotions. You are not these emotions. You can allow and make space for the feelings, but you don't have to lose yourself.

You are a bright light and your purpose here is to live a life of abundance and joy (even if it doesn't feel like it right now).

Part of every experience in life can all be part of your growth and evolution. It may be hard to see this when you are in pain. Every time I have had incredible pain in my life, I realized afterwards that it was something necessary for my progress and path in life. Some things we just can't make sense of with our minds and it is more of an acceptance from our hearts.

This final section is about moving forward and allowing yourself to dream and have desires. It's hard to do this if you are riddled with shame and guilt. I recommend you give that a lot of loving attention if it becomes impossible to move forward.

Many women choose to conceive again. Many women choose not to. Some women choose to adopt a child. This is unique and personal and can only come from you.

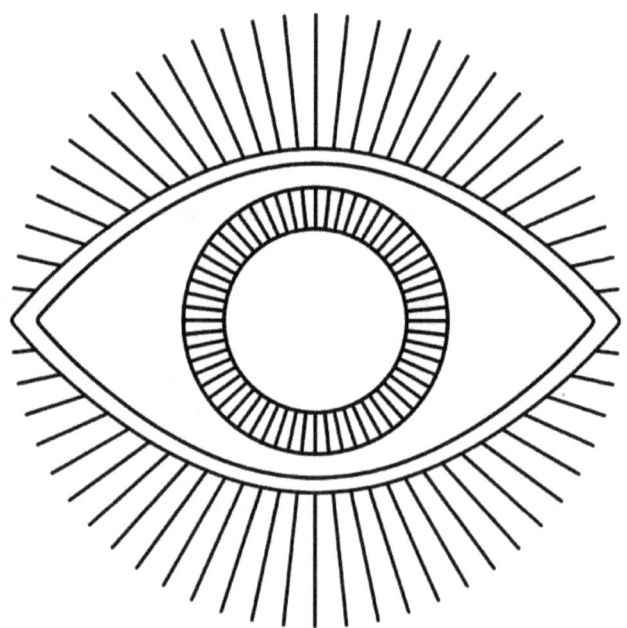

Journal Prompts

What is one way you can celebrate your lost baby's soul?

What feelings are you looking forward to? What feelings do you want to leave behind?

How can you make this week better than last?

Create a morning routine that would nurture and inspire you.

What does your ideal day look like?

What do you really desire for the future?

How do you see your happiest self? What is going on around you? Where are you? Who is with you?

What images bring feelings of joy?

Affirmations

I am grateful to be alive.

I let go of my sorrow, but will hold onto my love for my baby.

I am proud of who I am and the strengths that I have.

My intense pain means I am capable of so much love in the future.

I choose to see this as an opportunity for growth.

I can pay tribute to my baby by living in a beautiful way.

I deserve all the love, happiness and joy I desire.

It is safe to be all of me.

I create my life.

I go beyond fears and limitations of myself and others.

I can communicate with my heart and all is well.

I choose this life.

10

Conclusion

This is the end of the guide, but not the end of your journey. You may need to revisit sections of the book. Know that this is normal and it's all acceptable. The sections are not meant to be linear.

As stated earlier, grief is multi-faceted. Human beings are like onions. You peel back one layer and there are so many more layers. Let your intuition guide you to know what your body, mind, and soul needs most.

I do believe you are capable of feeling whole. You already are whole, even with this loss. It is possible to feel it again even if you don't believe it now. I will hold that faith for you.

Remember it is never too late to seek support from a friend, family member or seek help from a professional.

I hope you can use these tools to process and navigate your emotional experience, gain deep self awareness, and find comfort, strength and support within yourself.

If you enjoyed this book, please leave a favorable review on Amazon. I would appreciate that so much as I hope this book makes it into the hands of women who most need it and can be supported by it.

Know that I am here to support you as well. I have a passion for supporting women in life and I have the capacity to hold space for all of it. You can find out more about how to connect with me and the holistic, loving, deep support I provide through coaching at: www.heatheronhealth.com

I will end with a quote to inspire some peace and hope.

> "Those we love never truly leave us. There are things that death cannot touch." ~Jack Thorne

CONCLUSION

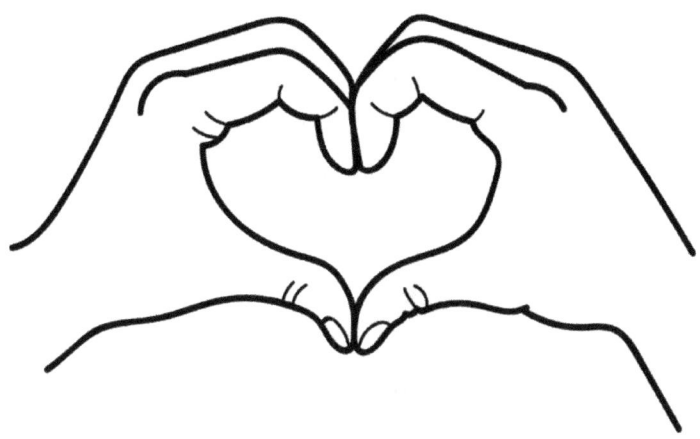

11

Resources

B. (2021, May 18). *100 Positive Affirmations For Mental Health*. Learning to Be Free. https://www.learningtobefree.com/2020/06/29/positive-affirmations-for-mental-health/

Barkley, S. (2022, March 9). *15 Mantras for Couples to Have a More Positive Marriage*. Power of Positivity: Positive Thinking & Attitude. https://www.powerofpositivity.com/positive-marriage-mantras/

Brock, F. (2019, August 28). *The Only 25 Affirmations You Need to Forgive Yourself*. Prolific Living. https://www.prolificliving.com/forgive-yourself-affirmations/

Cross, S. (2021, July 7). *A Ramble through Lamentation: Rituals for Expressing Grief*. Spirituality & Health. https://www.spiritualityhealth.com/articles/2020/07/06/a-ramble-through-lamentation-rituals-for-expressing-grief

EKR Foundation. (2020, July 8). *Elisabeth Kübler-Ross Biography*. https://www.ekrfoundation.org/elisabeth-kubler-ross/biography/

RESOURCES

Grabowski, S. (2022, March 21). *How To Use Affirmations To Reprogram The Subconscious Mind*. THE MINDFUL STEWARD. https://themindfulsteward.com/how-to-use-affirmations-to-reprogram-the-subconscious-mind/

One Life Counselling and Coaching. (2016, October 23). *5 Relationship Mantras to Transform Your Relationship | One Life Blog*. Www.Onelifecounsellingcoaching.Com. https://onelifecounsellingcoaching.com/blog/relationship-mantras-to-transform-relationships/

Rehman, A. L. (2022, January 7). *32 Journal Prompts for Grieving and Loss*. Grief Recovery Center. https://www.griefrecoveryhouston.com/journal-prompts-for-grieving-loss/

Smyth, J. M., Johnson, J. A., Auer, B. J., Lehman, E., Talamo, G., & Sciamanna, C. N. (2018). Online Positive Affect Journaling in the Improvement of Mental Distress and Well-Being in General Medical Patients With Elevated Anxiety Symptoms: A Preliminary Randomized Controlled Trial. *JMIR Mental Health*, 5(4), e11290. https://doi.org/10.2196/11290

Wagner, K. D. (2021, April 29). *16 Grief Affirmations for Coping With Loss*. Spirituality & Health. https://www.spiritualityhealth.com/articles/2016/08/22/16-affirmations-coping-grief

What Is Disenfranchised Grief? (2022, April 17). Verywell Mind. https://www.verywellmind.com/disenfranchised-grief-definition-causes-impact-and-coping-5221901

www.ingramcontent.com/pod-product-compliance
Lightning Source LLC
Chambersburg PA
CBHW060034040426
42333CB00042B/2437